The Family Guide to Nutrition and Fitness

Sheila Mattia Davtyan inspired by Adis Davtyan

ISBN:149741122X
ISBN-13:9781497411227

1

DEDICATION

We Dedicate this to Lulu and the future children.

Table of Contents

Chapter 1

A Call to Action

"If I knew I was going to live this long I would have taken better care of myself."

-Eubie Blake at age 100

As a parent you work hard every day to make sure your children have everything they need and much of what they want. If you could give your children a gift that would help them live longer and better lives would you give it to them? Of course you would.

Teaching your child how to make healthy eating and fitness a part of their everyday lives

6

will not only help them now, but will positively impact rest of their lives. They will have more energy, sleep better, feel better, and even think better. Chances are they will probably behave a little better too.

Pediatricians have heard it all. Toddlers who painstakingly find every pea in their meal and drop them meal and drop them off their highchair trays. Five-year-olds who sit on their sandwich and say "All done!" Tweens who use the old "Under the mashed potatoes" trick...as if we didn't do that ourselves when we were kids! Is it really worth the struggle to get children to eat a balanced diet?

Well, consider this. Kids who get to eat whatever they want will do just that. . . even if it makes them sick. Even if it makes them grumpy. Or listless. Or out of control. Kids aren't likely to connect a dinner of fries and purple ketchup with not being able to concentrate on homework later on....but you will.

The 'Food for the Brain' project found that when students' diets were positively modified there was as significant increase in their ability to concentrate, their behavior, and their academic performance. (Food for the Brain Staff)

The Center for Disease Control and Prevention says are society has become 'obesogenic' meaning America's cultural environment is such that it actually promotes an increase in food intake, unhealthy food choices, and physical inactivity. (Centers for Disease Control and Prevention, 2010) Our portions are larger, our hobbies are more sedentary, and are food choices are often quick and convenient rather than balanced and healthy.

` The only way to change this is one family at a time. As parents we must become advocates for our children's health by making a balanced diet and fitness an integral part of our family's everyday lives. The changes you make now will not only improve your children's lives, but will impact future generations as well. Just think, one day you will have healthier grandchildren because of the changes you make now!

We must work against all the negative messages our children are receiving in relation to nutrition and fitness. They are inundated with unhealthy images. Next time you watch a show with them on television help your children to keep a tally of how many healthy advertisements are shown versus how many unhealthy advertisements are shown. You may be quite shocked at your findings!

Our children's choices are manipulated from a young age. Of the food related commercials advertised on children's shows 70 percent advertise "junk" food. The statistics were even worse for our older children with 80% of MTV's food commercials advertising unhealthy food choices. (LiveScience Staff, 2009) These commercials definitely work on their target audience. Most children will ask for advertised products by name when at the grocery store rather than requesting healthy items. It is up to us to 'reprogram' them and teach them how to make healthy decisions for themselves.

So how do you improve your child's behavior, mood, and academic performance today—and reduce the likelihood of obesity, high blood pressure, diabetes, or heart disease tomorrow?

You fill your house with a variety of good foods—fruits, vegetables, whole grains, low-fat dairy products, lean meats, poultry, fish, beans, eggs, and nuts. Then, rather than battling over every Brussels sprout and bean, you get your children involved in planning and preparing meals. For kids, eating dishes they've helped create is completely different from insisting they eat foods that are "good for them."

The state of our youth is not just a personal problem, or even an isolated family problem. It is a national epidemic. Approximately 1.5 billion was spent last year on medical expenses associated with health issues attributed to being overweight or obese (Sloane, 2009). One in three American children is currently overweight and the heaviest percentage of those children are twice as likely to die early (before the age of 55) as their healthier classmates. (Rabin, 2010) To put it in better perspective look at the following comparison: there were approximately 400,000 preventable deaths last year associated with obesity (Fouad, 2004) compared to the 2,000 caused by the Swine Flu.

Eric Hartwell, British pediatrician says: Childhood obesity is one of the most important health issues in the world. More children are becoming dangerously overweight at an earlier age than ever before. Obesity brings with it the threat of numerous diseases, ranging from bone and joint problems to asthma and type 2 diabetes. On the brighter side, once a child begins to lose weight, these health problems seriously lessen or, in some cases, go away altogether.

Now let's look at some sobering statistics about *our nation's* children and the state of their health. Between 16 and 33 percent of kids are not just moderately overweight but obese. Weight issues usually begin between ages 5 and 6 or during early adolescence so now is the time to act on behalf of your child!

A child who struggles with obesity now, has an 80 percent chance of fighting with obesity for the rest of their lives. (American Academy of Child Adolescent Psychiatry, 2008) Unfortunately, obesity is not the only disease that our children will face if they enter adulthood without good physical and nutritional habits: diabetes, cardiovascular disease, and even asthma are all linked to childhood obesity. (Division of Nutrition, Physical Activity, and Obesity, 2009)

Unhealthy choices are causing our children to suffer from diseases that used to be issues associated with the middle aged or the elderly.

Even more worrisome is the psychosocial consequences often associated with being overweight. Children often suffer from negative body images and poor self-esteem that can adversely affect their interpersonal, social and academic lives. Studies have recently established that even if a child manages to lose weight in adulthood, some of the psychological damage from being an obese child linger. Obese children tend to have low self esteem and less confidence in social situations than their peers. Sometimes they will even try to avoid gym class out of shame for their appearance.

While obese children generally tend to have poor body images, this is not helped by all the teasing that they tend to have to endure at school and in other social situations with their peers. A lot of times, obese children will skip school or drop out altogether in order to avoid having to confront their peers' teasing and cruel remarks.

This psychological assault is why drug and alcohol use among overweight teenagers has also risen in recent years. Illicit substances have become an unfortunate way of escaping from and coping with the problem of obesity. Substance abuse problems also contribute to increasing the amount of depression an obese child suffers.

There are some things a parent can do to help lessen the psychological stress that results from obesity. You must confront the problem of overeating head on. Oftentimes, a child will overeat because they are depressed. Once this problem is brought out in to the open, it can be easier to find strategies for coping with it – not to mention alternative approaches to solving depression.

What's more, talk to your children about personal appearance and how they feel about themselves. Physical beauty is often dwelled on in this society to an unhealthy degree. Whatever happened to inner beauty? Highlight the qualities that make your child special – different, and thus more attractive to others.

Make it a daily habit to praise your children whenever they accomplish something positive.

It is important that when dealing with obesity in the family, you never use food as the basis of reward. When your child accomplishes something worth celebrating, splurge on a movie or another fun activity rather than fast food or eating out.

Children should never be criticized for not losing weight or accomplishing personal goals. Instead, the parent should always be constructive. Talk it out and find a solution.

Parents should also serve a good example for their kids. That means that the whole family should eat healthy and engage in physical activity as a unit. If you as a parent are not healthy on a mental and physical level, then you cannot expect your children to be, either.

Get your family moving! Inactivity has reached an all time high in our nation. Our kids and teens spend an average of four hours per day in front of the TV and two hours per day either on the computer or playing video games. This does not include the time they spend on the computer for homework. (Nemours Foundation, 2010) Between the eight hours a day they spend in school and the six hours they spend using electronics there is little time to fit any physical activity into their day. The sedentary lifestyle our young people have adopted may not have the immediate health issues that obesity does, but it will lead to significant health issues as they age. Many chronic illnesses can be curtailed by making just a few minor lifestyle changes now. Killers like heart disease, diabetes, colon cancer, high blood pressure, and obesity can be controlled through regular physical activity and a proper diet. (ASPE , 2002)

Studies have shown a positive link between children's' diet and exercise and their behavior. (Lehey, Maraget Ed.D. & Rosen, Shari, 2010) All parents have witnessed the effects of a 'sugar high' after a birthday party or holiday. Luckily, the after affects of too much sugar are short lived in instances like these. However, when a child's diet consistantly containes too much sugar or additives their behavior can be permanently modified. Symptoms resulting from a poor diet can include, irratibility, difficulty sleeping, trouble concentrating and hyperactivity. (David, 2000) Boys seem to be especially sensitive to additives in the foods they eat.

In response to the research experts are asking that synthetic dyes be banned in food marketed for children. As a parent we can't wait for others to make nutricional decisions for our children. We must be proactive in controlling what goes into our childen's stomachs.

Insufficient exercise can have similar negative effects on behavior just as unhealthy food choices can. Children often get in trouble at school due to behaviors like fighting, wiggling and disruptiveness. Often these disruptive behaviors stem from lack of exercise.

Conversely, childen who exercise regularly have more energy, sleep better, and pay better attention in school. They also have less anxiety and tension as exercise releases lactic acid from the blood. The production of endorphins produced when excercising helps create a sense of happiness and peace which in turn frees the mind to think better. (Ansorage, 2010)

Remember when your child was a baby or even a toddler? If they didn't get a good night's sleep the next they were miserable....as were you! Sleep is just as important for our older children. The National Sleep Foundation reccomends teens get a minimum of nine hours of sleep and elementary school age children get between ten and eleven hours of sleep. (NSF Staff, 2009) Lack of sleep resulting from poor diet or exercise can cause irritibility, memory loss, uncontrollable emotions, and social difficulties. It also hampers academic performance by decreasing attention span and making it difficult to recall or remember information.

A rundown body is easy prey for cold germs and viruses making sleepy children more succeptable to illnesses. Long term sleep deprivation has also been linked to depression and substance abuse in older children. Intrestingly, lack of sleep can also inadvertently cause weight gain as well. A tired brain gets its signals mixed up and thinks it is hungry when it is full. Sleep deprivation also causes the body to crave unhealthy foods. Proper fitness and nutrician help children sleep better which, in turn, improves many of the other areas of a child's life.

Eric Hartwell, British pediatrician says: "Childhood obesity is one of the most important health issues in the world". More children are becoming dangerously overweight at an earlier age than ever before. Obesity brings with it the threat of numerous diseases, ranging from bone and joint problems to asthma and type 2 diabetes. Once a child begins to lose weight, these health problems seriously lessen or, in some cases, go away altogether.

Now is the time for change. It will only get more difficult as your children get older. The habits your children develop now, both good and bad, will stick with them for the rest of their lives.

It is quite likely your children will be resistant to this change at first, especially your older ones. If you will stay firm and consistent they will gradually begin to see the benefits of healthy living. Chances are they will change their attitudes soon as they begin to see and feel the positive effects of your family's lifestyle change.

Chapter 2

Getting Started

"The best time to plant a tree was 20 years ago. The next best time is now."

-Chinese Proverb

Imagine your child was picked on everyday at school by a bully who stole from them and threatened their wellbeing. You would certainly take action immediately and do whatever it took to ensure your child's wellbeing. As parents we must view obesity and inactivity just as we would the very worst of schoolyard bullies. Right now is the time to take action. In this chapter we will look at how to get started.

While this book is aimed at how you can help your kids, a healthy and balanced lifestyle must become a family pursuit. Unless everyone is on board your children will most likely follow in your footsteps rather than listen to your words. Everybody purposes to eat better and to exercise more, but few follow through past the initial few attempts. There are all sorts of legitimate reasons for this: lack of time, lack of energy, and just not knowing how, are at the top of the list for most people.

If you are going to commit to healthy lifestyle changes the key is to find what works for your family. You must take your individual needs, schedule, and current lifestyle into consideration. Healthy eating and fitness become a part of your family's lifestyle, rather than take over your family's life. Moderation is the key. Telling your child they can never have treats can be just as damaging as continuously giving them treats. Healthy eating does not have to be complicated...just balanced!

It is very important to make everybody a part of the change. If your children are a part of this lifestyle change or shift, depending on where your family is starting from, they will be less likely to resist. Explain to them why you are making these changes as a family and respect their input.

Your very first step in a healthier lifestyle is to come up with a family action plan. Sit down (this is the only time in this book you will be advised to sit!) and write out short term and long term goals together. Short term goals are measured in weeks and months while long term goals are measured quarterly, bi-annually or even in years.

Each goal your family makes should be SMART: specific, measurable, achievable, relevant, and time bound. (Haughey, 2010) Consider working towards a long term goal that will benefit others as well as yourselves. Look ahead at upcoming walk-a-thons, runs and bike rides for various charities, and train specifically for that event as a family. Make sure to choose a cause that you feel strongly about. An achievable and important purpose will help keep you all motivated.

Experts recommend starting with between five and seven goals. This is a manageable place to start. Once you have completed writing your goals as a family post them in a common area where the whole family can see them. If your children enjoy art projects write the goals on poster board and let them color it and decorate it with stickers, and glitter. You may draw or add pictures next to the words if any of your children are too young to read.

Examples of SMART Goals

 Fitness Smart Goal Example: Our family will ride bikes on the local bike trail for 45 minutes after dinner each day in order to increase our cardiovascular endurance.

Long Term Fitness Smart Goal Example: In three months our family will ride in the yearly 10K cancer fundraiser on April 6th at 10:45.

Short Term Nutrition Smart Goal Example: Our family will cut our current soda intake down to one per day and substitute with water.

Long Term Nutrition Smart Goal Example: One month from today, April 2, 2010, we will no longer keep soda in the house. Soda consumption will be limited to dinners out and special occasions.

Chapter 3

Motivation

"Motivation is the electrical power that activates the engine of success."

-Ramez Sasson

I am sure you have heard the myth that it takes 21 days to form a habit, but that is only true for very basic habits like drinking a glass of water before bed. It takes an average of 66 days to form habits that involve lifestyle changes. (Dean, 2010)

So, the first few months your family embarks on a healthier and fitter lifestyle it will take a daily effort. Sometimes it will feel like an overwhelming task and it will take every bit of self-control you can muster to keep going. Remember if you quit, your children will too. Be firm, but instead of becoming a drill sergeant, use positive reinforcement.

To help keep everyone motivated you may want to set up a reward system. There are several ways to do this depending on the age of your children, the needs of your family and the amount of reinforcement you think they need. You may want to set up small weekly incentives as well as one large reward for after your family reaches each major milestone. You may purchase an incentive chart or checklist or make one the computer. Incentive charts can be bought at any teacher store and many office supply stores carry them as well.

For each day you meet your family goals let your children put a sticker or checkmark in the blank. At the end of each week use one of the recommended incentive ideas or create your own to keep everyone motivated: Celebrate, celebrate, and celebrate!

- **The Mystery Envelope:** Write down a list of several things your children enjoy doing or collecting on separate notecards and put each in a sealed envelope. Each week post one envelope next to the incentive chart. At the end of the week if the weekly goals have been met the children get to open up the envelope to see what the prize is for the week.

- **Wheel of Fortune:** Cut out a large circle on heavy cardboard or posterboard. Draw lines on it, so it looks like a wagon wheel when you are finished. On each triangle write a different incentive. For the spinner cut out an arrow and attach it to the center of the wheel with a brad. At the end of the week allow your child to spin to see what they win for the week.

- **Home Shopping Network:** Write a list of incentives on a poster in order of "price". Every day give your child an agreed upon amount of play money if they stick to the goals you have agreed upon without any arguing. If you have computer savvy children let them design your family's fun money using family pictures in the place of the presidents. Every Friday allow them to cash in to purchase one of the prizes. They may spend some of their money, all of their money or save up for a larger prize.

Allow your children to help you make a list of incentive ideas, so you are sure they will motivate them. You may be surprised with some of the things they think up! Incentives do not have to be expensive. Try to provide an even balance between event-oriented and prize-oriented motivators. Food in and of itself should never be a prize. but a family pizza night is perfectly acceptable. Let your budget and your time constraints be your guide.

For prizes keep an eye out for clearance items, art supplies, etc. to stash them away in your closet. Just make sure not to write anything down unless you can deliver it in a reasonable amount of time. A theme night should be honored within two or three days and gift incentives should be handed out immediately or they will lose their effectiveness.

Theme Ideas

Movie Night	Family Karaoke
Family Picnic	Backyard Camping

Arts and Crafts	Game Night
Slumber Party	Water Games
Game Night	Outdoor Game Day
Family Olympics	Make Your Own Pizza

Another way to stay motivated is to keep a record of your family's progress. Ask your children help chronicle your family's quest by making an online scrapbook, keeping a daily journal of your progress, or even make a video documentary. When the road gets rough look back at how far you all have already come and use that to motivate you to keep moving forward.

Keep in mind your goals should never focus on weight unless under the strict supervision of a physician. Healthy living is not about how much you weigh, but about eating smart and maintaining an active and balanced lifestyle. It is my recommendation that you do not even keep a scale in the house as your family begins this journey together. Make sure to revisit your goals every few months and make adjustments where needed. Don't forget to celebrate your successes every day!

Chapter 4

Nutritious Changes

"The first step toward change is awareness. The second is acceptance."

Nathaniel Branden

If your family is currently skipping meals, stop! It is important that everyone in your family eat three balanced meals a day. Skipping meals causes unhealthy cravings, low blood sugar and over compensation at the next meal.

Not surprisingly, Breakfast tends to be the most skipped meal of the day. Many people find themselves unable to eat early in the morning or just too rushed?

How often have you heard, "breakfast is the most important meal of the day"? Well, it bears repeating. A morning meal makes everything better—better energy, better concentration, better problem-solving skills, and better eye-hand coordination. That means better performance in school and a better appreciation and love for learning.

What's more, breakfast eaters tend to be healthier eaters overall, and these eating patterns usually continue into adulthood, helping people maintain a healthy weight and avoid heart disease and other serious health problems in the years ahead.

Granted, it's not always an easy task. Mornings are usually pretty hectic and getting a kid to eat more than a few bites before rushing to play or catch the bus is a challenge. But a few bites are better than nothing and you can work up from there.

Nowadays more and more schools are providing breakfast in an effort to boost academic performance and attendance and reduce behavior problems. These programs appear to be working—many schools report significant improvements, academically and socially.

So, what does a child typically eat for breakfast? It doesn't have to be fancy. In fact, there's growing evidence that a bowl of good old-fashioned oatmeal may be ideal. Several recent studies have shown that when kids eat oatmeal for breakfast— versus cold cereal or no breakfast at all—they have better memory and attention, skills that come in handy when studying subjects like math and geography.

Scientists think this effect is linked to whole-grain oatmeal's high-fiber, high-protein content. Because whole grains digest slowly, they supply the brain with a steady stream of energy.

Whether your child's favorite cereal is hot or cold, always check the nutrition label for fiber, protein, and sugar content per serving. At breakfast, you want to get plenty of fiber and protein into kids because it will keep them feeling full and energized until lunch. For the same reason, aim to keep sugar to a minimum; otherwise, it can send a kid's energy soaring up, then tumbling down before the morning's half over. In fact, sugar of any kind should not be among the first three ingredients on the label. What should be there:

- Fiber—at least 3 grams per serving; add a fistful of fresh fruit, raisins, dried cranberries, almonds, pecans, sunflower seeds, ground flax seed, or wheat germ, to bring the total to 6 grams

- Protein—at least 3 grams per serving
- Sugar—no more than 5 grams per serving

If your family is hooked on breakfast meats, opt for leaner ones, such as Canadian bacon, and/or limit them to once a week. Traditional breakfast meats tend to be high in saturated fat and/or sodium. You also can substitute chicken, turkey, or soy-based bacon and sausage.

Washing breakfast down with milk is a good choice for all age groups (though make it low-fat after age 2), and, while it shouldn't replace fresh fruit, 4 to 8 ounces of 100 percent juice per day is fine, too.

If your children have difficulties eating before school try giving them a smoothie to drink before they leave and send a breakfast bar (check the ingredients carefully. Many breakfast bars are just candy bars with better packaging.) with them for later on. You can pack much of the recommended dairy and fruit into a smoothie.

Now let's look at lunch. Does your child eat well-balanced, homemade lunches or school lunches?

A lot of parents prefer to give their kids a couple of dollars for a cafeteria lunch than make a brown-bag lunch assuming that a hot lunch is more nutritional than a bag lunch. The trouble is that school meals tend to sabotage children's eating habits.

Most school cafeterias still serve prepackaged, highly processed foods instead of whole grains, fresh fruits, and vegetables. In addition, you have no way of knowing if your child is skipping the entree and just eating cheese puffs and cookies. If junk food is available, kids will buy it. Studies show a direct link between the availability of junk food at school and a higher calorie and fat intake during school hours.

With a little planning, it is possible for your child to get a nutritious cafeteria lunch. Make a weekly date to review the school lunch menu together. Discuss what is offered and decide together what's best. It's a great opportunity to work through how to make healthy and tasty choices.

In general, however, bagged lunches are the best way to make sure your child eats healthy foods at school.

To see what they are and are not eating, ask younger kids to put their leftovers back into their lunch box, so you can see whether they ate that bag of baby carrots or the string cheese. It's a good way to judge what works at lunch time and what doesn't and talk about options. Also, getting kids involved in making their own healthy lunch the night before increases the odds that they'll actually eat it!

A word about cold cuts: You may find that your child wants to pack a bologna and cheese sandwich every day. Having one occasionally is fine, but processed meats are often high in saturated fat, sodium, and preservatives, and shouldn't be daily fare. Solution: Most grocery stores carry not only fresh turkey meat but also a variety of soy- and vegetable-based "deli meat" alternatives. Try them. You—and your kids—may be surprised by how good many brands are.

Give a child a choice between an apple and a box of candy and the apple will surely be tossed to the side. Children will always make the appealing choice rather than the healthy choice. As they eat the box of candy it quickly becomes evident that they do not know how to self regulate either. They will most likely polish off the box even if they start to feel sick to their stomachs. The ability to make healthy choices and self regulate are vital skills that children must be intentionally taught. They are best taught by proper modeling at mealtime as well as snack time.

Purposing to eat dinner together at the table as a family every night will help your children learn proper portions and help you keep an eye on what they are eating.   Regular family meals are also attributed to decreasing the risk of unhealthy weight control practices and substance abuse in teens. A Harvard study showed that children eat healthier when they share in family dinners.

How often do you sit down as a family and eat together? Ideally, seven days a week, but I know that isn't realistic. What with gymnastics on Mondays, soccer on Tuesdays, swimming on Thursdays—and your own book-group meetings on Fridays—sitting down together for dinner isn't always possible.

Still, try to schedule a family dinner several times a week, and some family breakfasts, too. Even kids who resist usually wind up enjoying getting parents' undivided attention to talk about their day. Making family meals a daily habit that children look forward to helps them develop healthier attitudes about food (and also discourages destructive weight-loss behaviors). With older children it is also a good way to make sure they are eating enough. Family meals help prevent and catch eating disorders like anorexia and bulimia.

Keep meals lively by ending with a joke or riddle to solve by the next meal. Keep conversation lively by purchasing a set of tabletop dinner cards. Each card has a different fun topic to discuss. Have everyone share something that went well or not so well that day. This routine helps build strong family relationships that last a lifetime.

Studies show that kids who sit down with their families have healthier attitudes toward food and eat more nutritious foods— if parents are a role model for good nutrition and eating habits. Key habits to establish (you'll benefit too!):

- Eating more slowly
- Chewing each bite and putting the fork down between bites
- Eating a variety of veggies every day
- Serving healthy portion sizes
- Drinking a tall glass of water or milk instead of soda

Kids who eat while watching TV— even educational programs—tend to eat fewer fruits and vegetables, more snack foods and sodas, and more calories, probably because they focus on what they're watching, not what they're eating. Sound familiar?

Okay, you've managed to turn off the TV and your family is sitting down to a nutritionally rich, balanced, and tasty meal that the kids helped you plan, shop for, and prepare. Should you make them clean their plates?

No. The "clean plate club" is an old-fashioned notion that deserves to be thrown out the window. Forcing kids to eat even when they're full will not only ruin dinner but can nurture an overeater and lead to weight problems later in life.

Your child should learn to recognize what fullness feels like and know when to stop eating. If you're worried about wasting food, just serve children realistic portions. If it's not enough, they can always get a second helping.

Desert Anyone?

Make dessert an exception, not the rule, and not a reward for eating every bite. Children seem to have a natural inclination toward sweets. And as they grow, so does their sweet tooth.

Although totally restricting processed sweets may be the healthiest option, it might not be the smartest one. Studies have found that exerting too much diet control can backfire—kids who aren't allowed any treats tend to overindulge at the first chance or obsess about forbidden foods. So allow a couple of cookies after dinner once or twice a week and chocolate cake on birthdays.

After all, it's not the occasional sugar-filled treat that's detrimental, it's a steady diet of sweets. To satisfy their sweet tooth offer "desserts" like watermelon, or yogurt, granola, and fruit parfaits instead!

For meal time remember, healthy eating does not have to be complicated. When cooking meat don't fry it if you can bake it, steam it or grill it. Season foods as you cook them, keeping salt, pepper and butter off of the table. If you do not have time to cook pick up a roast chicken and a prepackaged salad from the grocery store on your way home instead of fast food.

As far as meats and poultry go, which types does your child eat fairly regularly?

Beef, pork, lamb, and poultry have long been a staple of family dinners. All provide complete protein, which means they contain the nine essential amino acids the body can't make on its own. These amino acids help build muscle cells, immune cells, blood cells, enzymes, and other structures.

Consuming enough protein also has been shown to enhance learning and intellectual development. Not only that, the zinc found in chicken, pork, and beef is beneficial to a healthy immune system. Likewise, the linoleic acid in meat may help prevent certain diseases, such as arthritis, breast cancer, and eczema.

However, since red meat is also a major source of saturated fat and cholesterol, choose wisely. What's best? It depends. Fat content varies with cut and grade. For example, white meat chicken is lower in fat than dark, and round and loin cuts of beef and pork are the most lean. Also, trimming off most visible fat before cooking significantly reduces the amount of saturated fat you eat, as does removing the skin on poultry.

Fishing anyone? Although often not a favorite with kids, fish is perhaps the most beneficial protein food. It contains the high-protein pluses of meat minus the saturated fat found in beef, pork, and poultry. Instead, it has important heart-healthy omega-3 fatty acids. Good omega-3 fats decrease risky triglycerides, inhibit damaging inflammation, help keep arteries clear, and improve blood vessel function. So try to work seafood—salmon, canned light tuna, oysters, herring, and cod—into your family's menu.

According to recent research, even eating fish as seldom as three times per month can have a beneficial effect. A good way to ensure your family eats enough seafood is to make grocery day seafood day. Buy one fresh, on-sale item from the seafood department of your grocery store when you do your weekly shopping and eat it that night.

Mealtimes should be balanced. Don't just serve the foods you know your child already likes. It's like school: Your child is constantly exploring new subjects there. You want him to constantly be learning about new foods at home. This will pave the way for a lifetime of better moods and better health.

Encourage your children to eat a little bit of everything across the food groups rather than a lot of one thing. Teach them to stop eating when they are no longer hungry rather than stuffing themselves or eating everything on their plate. Don't worry about the balance of your child's diet in a single meal. Think about it in terms of a week. Focusing on broader patterns is a much more constructive approach.

Keep in mind that all kids go through stages. At times, they will honestly not be hungry. Usually, this happens in a dormant phase of their growth cycle and it's okay for them not to eat much then. Just brace yourself: The next thing you know, they'll be ravenous and you won't be able to keep enough food in the house.

How do you know if kids are eating too much? Easy: They gain extra weight. Your pediatrician can help you determine what weight is normal for your child and what's not. Again, depending on growth spurts and activity levels, the amount kids eat can vary a lot. What seems like too much to you might be just what their growing bodies need at the time. If the food is healthy, most kids will eat till they are disinterested or distracted, which usually means they are full. On the other hand, if you're worried that your child isn't eating enough, keep in mind that compared with adult servings, a child's serving is pretty small. For instance, a toddler-sized portion may be just a couple of tablespoons.

When the Cornell Food Lab asked study participants from Paris and Chicago, "How do you know when you are through eating dinner?" To find out how Parisians can eat so well and still have much lower incidences of obesity and heart disease, they found the Parisians relied on internal cues to tell then when they were done. They stopped eating when they no longer felt hungry, when the food stopped tasting good, or in time so still have room for dessert. Americans relied on external clues. They felt they were done eating when their plate was clean, their television show was over, or the others at the table were finished. (Wansink, 2008).

Young children—under age 4—generally eat till they're not hungry, then stop. However, as kids get older, they tend to start ignoring their internal hunger cues and eat according to other influences, such as the amount of food on their plate. Studies show that serving children larger portions encourages them to eat more.

So rather than dishing out a lot of food, start with small servings, and use small, lunch-sized plates rather than dinner plates so meals don't look skimpy. Then, offer seconds if your child is still hungry. One of the keys to maintaining a healthy relationship with food is learning how to gauge internal hunger cues.

Also, serve water with meals, not sugared or carbonated drinks, and encourage kids to take their time when eating. It takes about twenty minutes for the brain to register that the stomach is full, so overeating is frequently the result of eating too fast. Finally, let go of the notion that meals end with dessert, unless it's fruit.

Unfortunately, while kids today are getting enough calories—often more than enough—too few of these calories are coming from nutritionally sound sources. A recent study of 2- to 11-year-olds showed that about one-third of them were not meeting the daily requirements for fruits, grains, meats, dairy products, and vegetables. Perhaps most surprising, 16 percent did not meet any of the recommendations at all! So, where are kids' calories coming from? You guessed it: fats and sugars—two things that should be playing minor roles in their diets.

Filling up on "junk," such as chips, cookies, and soft drinks, usually means that protein, fiber, healthy fats, and essential vitamins and minerals get pushed out. The result over time: A greater risk for a number of health problems, including obesity, heart disease, and diabetes, just to name a few.

That's not to say that fat should be eliminated from a child's diet. Actually, during the early childhood years, kids need dietary fat for proper growth and neurological development. Fat also helps the body absorb certain nutrients and is necessary for maintaining energy levels. But fat should come from nutritious foods such as nuts, avocados, olive and vegetable oils, and low-fat dairy products (yogurt, cheese, and milk). Until the age of 2, children need whole-fat dairy products; after that, switching to lower-fat options is generally acceptable. Fat should make up a little less than a third of your child's diet. However, because individual needs vary, discuss this with your child's pediatrician.

Ready for snack time? What are typical snacks for your child? Somewhere along the line, snacks got a bad rap. Perhaps it was the constant warning, "No snacking between meals, you'll spoil your dinner!" Certainly, munching on too many cookies can cause kids to lose their appetite for meals.

You will often hear people attribute unhealthy weights with snacking. However, when chosen wisely, snacks provide another opportunity for kids to get the nutrients they need. Young kids need smaller portions of food more often since their stomachs are pretty small. The trick is to make sure that snacks pack as much nutritional punch and fiber as possible without a lot of saturated fat and calories.

So, while the choice and amount of snacks can be unhealthy, there is nothing wrong with savvy snacking as long as it does not interfere with mealtime. Many experts recommend light snacks between meals. Small snacks also can be an effective way to prevent overeating; they stave off excessive hunger, so kids don't become ravenous and reach for junk food. On the other hand, children should not be snacking so much that they're not hungry for meals. Establishing set snack times will also help fight emotional eating—snacking because of boredom or stress. Plan snack times after school or half way between meals or bedtime and prepare them for your children to limit quantities and insure quality.

Think about placement. Make it as easy as possible for your child to reach for that cut-up fruit and yogurt instead of chocolate-chip cookies. If healthy snacks are more convenient, you'll encourage healthy snacking habits. If your children are home alone in the afternoons create a shelf in the pantry and in the fridge where you place kid friendly snacks they are allowed to have. Try adapting a strategy from grocery stores: put the food you want to "move" where your "customers" can't miss it. Always keep fresh fruit on the counter where it's easy to grab and place veggies at the front and center of the refrigerator. That way when kids get the urge to munch, they'll be more likely to reach for a peach or some pea pods and carrots, especially if they are already cut up. If you're pressed for time, buy packaged, ready-to-go fruits and veggies. It might cost more, but it's cheaper than a box of cookies—or filling a cavity.

Teach your children to avoid eating food out of a bag or box. Instead place handful or two on a plate and then put the rest away...and no going back for more! According to a Cornell University study, when moviegoers were given large tubs of stale popcorn they ate 34 percent more than those given stale popcorn in medium sized containers. Ewww! This implies that portion size can lead to overeating just because it is available.

Keep food in the kitchen or at the table. If you limit where your children are allowed to eat they will be more likely to eat only when they are hungry and not out of habit, compulsion or boredom. Of course there will be exceptions, like popcorn on movie nights, but overall try to adhere to this rule. Not only is it better for your children it is better for your couch as well!

Chapter 5

Finding Time to Eat Right

"To eat is a necessity, but to

eat intelligent is an art"

-La Rochefoucauld

One of the things that often stands in the way of getting healthy is the busyness of life. It is very difficult to find the time to research healthy recipes, check the labels at the grocery store, and prepare a meal worthy of the Food Network when you are balancing work, a family, and daily life. Our kids usually prefer the instant food anyway. It is always disheartening when you spend thirty minutes making real macaroni and cheese and your family informs you they like the stuff out of the box better!

Food is good medicine; each group contains hundreds of unique and powerful substances that promote good health. While getting an appropriate amount of each major kind of food every day is a good start, in order to make your child's diet really work, you need to tap the wide range of nutrient-rich foods within each group.

It is an urban myth that it takes a lot less time to throw an instant meal in the oven or microwave than to cook a healthy dinner from scratch. It just takes a little preparation on the frontend.

Take the time to plan out a menu for the next week or for two weeks before you go shopping. Put the menu on the fridge and stick to it. Make sure to give yourself one, "Get out of the kitchen free" card a week for when you have one of those absolutely exhausting or extra busy days.

Choose one day a week, preferably a day off to be your prep day. Do what you can to get what you can ready for the week ahead. For example, if you buy a pack of chicken breasts cook them all on your day off, let's say Sunday. Once they are cooked chop them up. You can make three different meals out of them during the course of the week. You can make a chicken stir fry, a Greek chicken salad, and chicken fajitas, all of which can be made in less than 10 minutes, since the meat is already made.

Cut up any vegetables you will need for the week. Label them and place them in storage containers so they are ready when you need them. Make a large fruit salad to have on hand for breakfast, lunches or snacks throughout the week. Always make a big enough meal on Sunday to last for two days since Monday is always a tough day.

For evenings that you know you will be rushed, like sports practice nights, church, etc. Cook a big meal that will give you enough food for two nights the day prior or throw something in the slow cooker before you leave in the morning.

Another golden rule is to always make double. anytime you make anything big like vegetable lasagna, turkey meatballs or a casserole for example, make two and freeze one for later. It takes about the same amount of time to make one as it does to make two, plus you cut clean up in half. Those new throw away pans are great for this! Just put a freezer bag over them and toss them in the freezer. Then just pull them out to defrost the night before you need them. When you are done...throw away the pan. No clean-up! Every extra second counts during a busy work week.

Always keep at least three or four staples for quick and healthy meals in your pantry or freezer as a back-up. This will keep you from rushing to the phone to order out on days you just can't cook. Healthy soups as well as various whole grain pastas and tomato sauces are always good to have on hand for a quick meal.

Finally, get to know the menus of your favorite restaurants and choose smart meals when you do choose to eat out.

Let's look at how this would look in a typical week.

Sunday: Approximate time needed: 1 Hour

1. Cook chicken breast and chop it up. Separate it into three containers.
2. Chop up vegetables needed for the week. Place in separate containers and label.
3. Cut up vegetables for snacks and lunches for the week.
4. Make a large fruit salad for snacks, breakfast, and lunch for the week.
5. Cook a large meal like vegetable lasagna. Make two and freeze one for later.

Monday's Dinner: Eat leftover vegetable lasagna from Sunday's meal. Make a spinach salad to go with it. Slice Italian bread into extra thin slices and spread with mix of crushed garlic, olive oil and your family's preferred spices.

Tuesday's Dinner: Chicken and Vegetable Stir Fry. Start your rice or noodles. Stir Fry your vegetables in low sodium soy sauce and then add the chicken to heat it up. Put everything over the finished noodles or rice.

Wednesday' Dinner: Put a roast in the slow cooker along with vegetables. When you come home from work throw some whole grain biscuits in the oven and you are done.

Thursday's Dinner: Place salad in a bowl and add the cut up vegetables, chicken, and feta cheese. Add just a bit of Greek salad dressing. Serve with low-carb warm whole wheat pita bread.

Friday: Make pizza as a family instead of ordering them out. Use a whole wheat thin crust for your base. Let your children put the sauce and cheese on. Then put the vegetables you chopped for pizza on Sunday out for your children to choose from as well as any meat toppings.

Saturday: Sautee vegetables for fajitas and throw in the chopped chicken at the end to warm it up. Heat up tortillas and serve.

It is that simple. Your week is done, your family has eaten smart, and you have spent minimal time in the kitchen!

What If Your Child Wants to Become a Vegetarian?

What would you do if your child suddenly decided to become a vegetarian or vegan? If you're a meat eater, you'd worry, right? About whether she'll get all the nutrients she needs if she cuts out foods you believe are essential? You might even attempt to forbid it, or dismiss it as a youthful whim.

For most kids, the decision to become a vegetarian or vegan is a thoughtful one, based on ethical concerns about animals and the planet, or health issues, or both. Even if it seems to be just a phase or an assertion of independence, this lifestyle choice deserves respect and support.

First, you need to determine how far she plans to go in excluding certain foods:

- Lacto-ovo vegetarians eat eggs and dairy products.
- Ovo vegetarians eat eggs but no dairy.
- Vegans don't eat foods that are derived from any animal source, so eggs and dairy are not included. Because vegan diets are so restrictive, it can be difficult to meet the nutritional and caloric needs of a growing child.

Educating yourself and your child about this way of eating is critical. You must provide alternatives for foods that have been eliminated, and be sure that your novice vegetarian is getting enough of the vital nutrients needed for overall health.

The major concern is protein. But by pairing certain foods, your child can get the total protein that is found in meat. For instance, combining either legumes (e.g., beans, lentils) with whole grains or seeds, or dairy products with grains, creates a complete protein. Eggs also contain complete protein, but don't rely on them exclusively.

If your child "goes vegan"—that is, eliminates all animal products, including milk, eggs, and cheese—encourage her to eat plenty of fresh, dark green veggies for iron, B vitamins, and other minerals, and to drink soy milk fortified with vitamin B12 and calcium. Soy- and other vegetable-based meat alternatives are now widely available, so stock your freezer with these healthy protein sources.

Chapter 6

Savvy Shopping

"Grocery shopping with children is like being pecked to death by ducks".

-Author Unknown

How many times per month does your child participate in choosing healthy foods for dinner? Good nutritional habits come from more than just eating. Kids should also be involved in the selection, preparation, and presentation of meals. It's the best way to teach them about healthy food. You can start as early as age 3 with activities such as adding dry ingredients to a mixing bowl and helping to choose foods at the grocery store.

Yes, it can be a hassle to take kids to the supermarket. They squirm in the cart or disappear down the aisle; they get bored, bicker, and ask for all kinds of tempting junk food. You'd probably rather leave them at home. But if you do, your kids won't learn how to shop smart, and that's a lesson they can't afford to miss. So try some of these shopping tips:

- Be a taskmaster. Give each child a job to do—finding items on the shopping list or wrapping the twist ties around the produce bags. Older kids can manage coupons. Keep them busy, and they'll have less time to pester each other, and you.

- Celebrate something old, something new. To help get a wide variety of healthy foods into the family diet, let each child select an old favorite and then pick out something that they've never tried before.

- Let teens be chef for a day. Have them choose a recipe ahead of time and then put them in charge of collecting the ingredients and preparing the dish for the family to try.

- Make a game of it. Tell young children that the family is going to eat a rainbow, and have them choose fruits and vegetables from every color group.

- Bring munchies. Pack a snack to keep children happy, not hungry and cranky, while shopping.

- Put them in control. If your children are old enough to maneuver a kid-sized cart around the store, give them five items to find for their cart. Just be sure to teach them the rules of the road first!

- Give 'em label lessons. Teach your kids how to compare labels. For example, have them check a few different loaves to find the one with the most fiber. Showing children why certain foods are better than others will benefit their health for years to come.

Giving kids the power to make some decisions about food makes healthy eating easier and more enjoyable for everyone.

Important Safety Note: A stunning 24,000 kids wound up in the ER in 2006 as a result of shopping-cart accidents. If possible, don't put your child in a front-basket seat. Instead, look for carts with molded low-down child seats attached to them (these often look like cars). They are far safer than regular wire carts. And never put infant carriers on top of a shopping cart. Instead, use one of those strap-on chest carriers that holds your baby against your body, leaving your arms free.

No one has time to scrutinize every item they purchase at the grocery store, but there are a few basic rules that can help you make healthy choices as you shop. The following ingredients are best to stay away from completely: partially hydrogenated oils, saturated fats, dyes, trans fats, high fructose corn syrup, and refined sugars. With that in mind, you vow to buy all the "reduced-fat," "no-fat," "low carb," "less sugar," and "all natural" snacks you can find. Hold on a minute. Turn the package over and read the ingredients label.

The ingredients are listed in descending order, by weight. That means the first ingredients play a starring role in the snack you choose for your child. If flour is listed, look for whole grains. They offer many health benefits, including complex carbohydrates, which are healthier because they take longer to digest and help control blood sugar levels.

Be aware that just because something lists "wheat" flour doesn't mean that it's whole wheat. And enriched flour is refined flour that has nutrients added back in. Why take them out in the first place?

Stay away from foods that contain trans fats, which are also listed as hydrogenated or partially hydrogenated oil. Cookies, crackers, icing, potato chips, margarine, and microwave popcorn often contain these fats.

Trans fats are made using a process called hydrogenation that turns unsaturated fats into highly stable saturated fats that resist turning rancid. About twenty years ago, manufacturers began putting trans fats into processed foods to extend their shelf life. However, it turned out that these man-made fats are much riskier than any natural fat, even the saturated fats found in butter, beef, and pork. Several studies have found that trans fats raise the risk of heart disease, increase total cholesterol, and reduce healthy HDL good cholesterol.

Your body does need some fat, so don't avoid it alltogether. Just concentrate on the heart-healthy fats found in plant-based foods—nuts, avocados, olive oil, flaxseed and sesame oils, and more.

I am sure you have heard the phrase, "Less is more" many times. In the case of fruits and vegetables this is certainty the case! When you are food shopping the less ingredients a food product has the better it probably is for you! When you buy fruits and vegetables always buy fresh when possible. Try to buy a vast array of colors. A good goal is to try to buy a fruit and a vegetable for each of the colors of the rainbow. This ensures they will get a wide array of antioxidants, vitamins and minerals. If you must buy frozen produce buy it without any added sugar, seasonings or added ingredients like sauce or cheese. It is better to add those yourself in *very* limited quantities.

When buying prepackaged goods look for the words 'all natural' on the label when you are shopping. All natural peanut butter tastes just as good, but doesn't have the hydrogenated oils or sugars regular peanut butter does. Spreadable fruit just has fruit instead of the excess sugars and other additives that jelly has.

Let's talk about beverages next. What does your child drink most often?

Liquids do more than just quench kids' thirst. Beverages replace the liquid their bodies lose through activity and normal body function and, when chosen wisely, can also provide a nutritional boost. So make sure your child's beverages count.

Plain old water is best for keeping small bodies hydrated and functioning at their best, but other drinks, such as low-fat milk and 100 percent juice, can be a good way to fill in nutritional holes. Steering kids toward these beverages and away from sugar- or caffeine-filled drinks can help them maintain a healthy weight and healthy smile for years to come.

If you're not able to breastfeed for the entire first year of your baby's life, as the American Academy of Pediatrics recommends, be assured that even nursing for a few weeks gives your newborn some nutritional and immune-system benefits. If you stop breastfeeding before one year, switch to iron-fortified formula, not cow's milk. Your pediatrician can guide you in selecting one that is just right for your baby.

It is important to optimize bone health early on. Think of bone as a savings account; kids' bodies constantly make deposits and withdrawals of bone tissue. During childhood and adolescence, more bone is deposited than withdrawn as the skeleton grows in both size and density. A diet rich in calcium and other minerals keeps withdrawals, or bone loss, to a minimum. Kids with the highest peak bone mass after adolescence have the greatest advantage in terms of future bone health. So optimizing bone health early in life is crucial in preventing future fractures and osteoporosis. Soda, alcohol, high caffeine consumption, certain medications, antacids that contain aluminum, calorie restriction, and a lack of exercise are some common causes of low bone density.

If your child doesn't drink milk or eat any other high-calcium foods, such as yogurt, cheese, or calcium-fortified orange juice, then taking a multivitamin containing vitamin D and a calcium supplement is essential.

Since few children consistently meet the recommended intake of fruits and vegetables, sipping a moderate amount of 100 percent juice is one way to fill in some of their nutrient gaps. Juice is a great source of vitamin C and is often fortified with calcium. And because it's on the sweet side, even the pickiest of children enjoy it. What's more, several products now contain both fruit and vegetable juice, including Vruit, Odwalla, V8 V.Fusion, and Juice Plus, among others.

The key with juice is to sip, not guzzle. Be wary of allowing your child to fill up on juice— there may not be room left for the other foods needed for a well-balanced diet. Also, juices often are high in simple sugars and calories, which promote tooth decay and weight gain. They also lack the fiber and full nutritional punch of whole fruits and vegetables, so they're not a full replacement for these foods. For example, whole apples are high in protective phytochemicals that may help reduce the risk of certain types of cancer, asthma, diabetes, and cardiovascular disease. Apple juice isn't.

The importance of kids staying hydrated during intense physical activity is often overlooked. The more vigorous the activity, or the warmer the weather, the more critical it is for them to take in enough fluids. Talk with kids about how often and how much they should be drinking.

Often children are too busy having fun to notice internal or external cues telling them they are thirsty or becoming dehydrated. The amount of fluids needed will vary from child to child, so teach kids to pay attention to signs that they may be getting a little dehydrated, such as their lips being dry or their mouth feeling gummy or sticky. With increased dehydration comes shakiness, headaches, and stomachaches.

Water is the best choice for overall hydration, unless you've got a superactive kid. Your child may prefer sports drinks like Gatorade or Propel, but some sports drinks contain caffeine and many have high-fructose corn syrup—which will add to your kid's daily calorie intake and has some worrisome side effects.

Many experts partly blame the dramatic increase in childhood obesity on the overconsumption of sweetened soft drinks such as soda, iced tea, punch, and artificially flavored fruit beverages. A single 12-ounce can of these has as much as 13 teaspoons of sugar in the form of high-fructose corn syrup (HFCS). This thick liquid is made from cornstarch and, unlike other sweeteners, it disrupts the body's production of certain hormones that help regulate appetite and fat storage. As a result, some nutrition experts believe that HFCS-sweetened beverages throw off the body's normal weight-regulating mechanisms.

That means kids get a bunch of empty calories that leave their bodies craving even more calories. A recent study revealed that drinking one can of sugary soda a day increases their risk of becoming obese by 60 percent!

As for young teeth, sodas are doubly destructive because their sugar promotes decay, while their acidity destroys protective enamel— even in sugar-free sodas. In addition, adolescents, who need more than double the calcium of young children, are increasingly choosing soda over milk, which puts their bone development and overall healthy growth in jeopardy.

It is best to limit beverages to milk and water. Sodas should be eliminated all together, Think of Sodas as liquid candy. They add an enormous amount of calories and provide no nutritional value whatsoever. In addition they can cause or contribute to health problems like tooth decay, weaker bones, kidney stones, dehydration, blood sugar disorders and obesity. (Healthy Child Staff, 2010) Diet sodas are no better. It is best to keep them out of the house and allow soda only on special occasions like when out to dinner or at a party.

The fruit and vegetable blends are your best bet when it comes to juices. Keep other juices to an absolute minimum. Instead, keep your fridge stocked with bottled water to encourage your children to drink it instead.

Organic foods are very expensive so how do you decide what is worth paying the extra money for? Research by the Environmental Working Group says you can reduce pesticide exposure by 90% by buying organics of the following food: apples, bell peppers, celery, cherries, grapes, lettuce, nectarines, peaches, pears, potatoes, spinach, and strawberries. They also recommend buying organic eggs, meat, poultry, dairy, baby food and rice if possible. Keep those fruits listed in mind when buying juices as well.

When buying snacks remember your children will not eat it if you don't have it in the house. Make an effort to make every calorie count and replace unhealthy favorites with more nutritious alternatives. Buy chewy granola bars instead of candy bars, salsa and tortilla chips can replace chips and dip, and many of the sweeter cereals are now made with whole grain and packed with vitamins. Cereals make a nutritious nighttime snack.

Make healthy eating easy and keep healthy snacks accessible. Busy lifestyles often mean grabbing whatever is most convenient when you are in need of a snack. Keep items like fresh fruit, cheese sticks, nuts, and cut up vegetables cut up, ready to eat and visible.

To introduce more foods into a kid's diet, don't try to revamp the family's eating habits overnight. First tackle the excesses and then focus on the deficiencies. Modest changes are more likely to add up to positive, lifelong eating habits.

Try to slowly expand the menu by focusing on what we call the three Ts: tint (color), texture, and taste. You can't go wrong if you have a good variety of these on the plate. Here's why:

- Tint—The more colorful the mix of food on the plate, the greater the nutritional payoff. Richly colored fruits and veggies— bright berries, sunny tangerines, emerald spinach, red bell peppers—contain important protective phytochemicals and antioxidants that help prevent disease and preserve health in many ways. They also can help cool inflammatory activity in the body that, among other things, contributes to heart and blood vessel disease. When kids are young, try making weekly fruit and vegetable charts together, and have your child place a star for each vegetable or fruit eaten. Hang it on the refrigerator for inspiration.

Allow a little more time than usual on your next grocery run. When you hit the produce aisle, focus more on the colors than on specific foods. Use this grocery list to help you explore.

- Texture—Keep things crunchy with veggies, whole grains, seeds, and nuts. All are nutritional powerhouses and many are filled with insoluble fiber, which helps ward off type 2 diabetes and works to keep your child's colon healthy by helping intestinal function. Insoluble fiber is mainly found in whole grains like oats, barley, brown rice, whole-wheat breads and pasta, and whole-grain breakfast cereals, but veggies like carrots, zucchini, celery, Brussels sprouts, cabbage, and cauliflower are packed with it, too. Sunflower, sesame, and pumpkin seeds are healthy sources of vitamins, minerals, protein, amino acids, and good (unsaturated) fats, so sprinkle them on main dishes, salads, and sandwiches. The same goes for nuts such as cashews, almonds, walnuts, pecans, and pine nuts.

- Taste—Introduce your child to new flavors by cooking with different herbs, spices, and sauces. With stronger flavors (ginger, dill, horseradish), use a light hand at first. Some will fly, some won't—for now—but every bit of progress counts.

Applying this 3-Ts strategy to family meals will help ensure that your child has the right balance of calories, proteins, minerals, and vitamins—not only for healthy physical growth but also for proper brain development, weight control, disease prevention, and more.

Chapter 7

All Aboard!

"Individual commitment to a group effort- that is what makes a team work, a company work, a society work, a civilization work."

-Vince Lombardi

The hardest thing about getting your family on a healthier course is getting

everybody to make the commitment. It can take a lot of convincing and perhaps some pleading and bribery as well! On the other hand if you make it fun your children might jump on the healthy bandwagon quicker than you think.

Teach your children how to look at labels to check for quality ingredients and the importance of comparing products. (Please do not teach them to check calories; which puts the emphasis on weight rather than healthy eating.) Let your children help plan the weekly menu, cut coupons and go grocery shopping with you. Go to the local farmer's market together, visit a self-pick farm or plant a family garden. Make healthy eating an adventure!

How about meal preparation—does your child help out? Kids tend to get overexcited right before dinnertime. They've had some downtime from school, done their homework, and may be anxious for a parent to arrive home from work.

This is a great time to focus their energy on helping with the meal.

Even toddlers can be given a job to do—something as simple as putting napkins on the table. Older kids can stir sauces or, with supervision, chop vegetables. Teenagers who like to cook can prepare a whole dish or even a whole meal once a week.

Make sure the task is age-appropriate (no sharp or pointed utensils for little ones). Thank them for their efforts and overlook the less-than-perfect. Who cares if a recipe doesn't turn out perfectly, or a little milk is spilled in the pouring? Keep the goal in mind: family fun and healthy habits.

Making meal preparation a family activity has multiple rewards. You'll find that putting kids in charge of a few things makes them more likely to enjoy mealtimes together. It also makes cooking less of a chore for you, so you're more likely to make a homemade meal rather than dialing out for pizza again (which is allowed sometimes, too!). Plus, kids are more likely to eat dishes— even unusual ones—they helped create.

Cook meals together as a family as much as possible. Children are much less resistant to new foods when they have helped choose them and prepare them. Many popular chefs have written children's cookbooks as well. Invest in a few of their favorites and let them pick one healthy recipe a week to cook on their own or with moderate assistance depending on their age.

Make a big deal about healthy cooking. Buy your children their own colorful measuring cups and spoons. Buy plain aprons and puffy paint at your local craft store and let your children decorate their own aprons. Get everyone in the kitchen when it is time to cook. Put some music on and have some family fun!

You can also get creative. Start some meal time traditions. Have a weekly pizza night and let your children choose their toppings and make their own personal pan pizzas. A monthly international night can inspire your children to try new foods. Choose a country or region and research and cook healthy recipes from the area. You can expand on this and make a whole night of it. Decorate your dining room and play traditional games from the country, make crafts, and learn some words or phrases in their language. Host an Iron Chef cook-off. Break the family into teams and give each team the same healthy ingredients to create a meal with. You may be surprised at what they come up with!

Chapter 8

Fitness Basics

"An hour of basketball feels like 15 minutes. An hour on a treadmill feels like a weekend in traffic school."

-David Walters

Inactivity has become a national issue. In response to this, President Obama has initiated a challenge to all Americans. The Presidents

Challenge asks each and every family to choose an activity, get active for 60 minutes a day, and track your activity. This goal of his challenge is to help Americans get started down the road towards a healthier lifestyle. Notice the wording of the challenge. He did not say run for sixty minutes or do sit-ups for 60 minutes. The challenge is simply to get active. It does not have to be a torturous event. That means your family can do whatever they want for the 60 minutes as long as they are up and moving. You do not need to train for a triathlon, but simply make fitness a part of your family's daily routine. It can be as simple as walking every day after dinner.

Fitness should not be repetitive and boring. Make fitness fun and let your family's interests drives your activities. If your children love to ride bikes, then go for a bike ride after dinner every day. If they love to play soccer then play soccer in the backyard as a family. If your children do not have any preferences then have fun trying out new things together until you find some activities everybody enjoys. Be creative: Kayaking, Yoga, Frisbee-golf, hiking, spelunking....the list is endless.

If you live in a location where outdoor activities are not an option much of the year you may consider joining a local gym together that focuses on the needs of families. The YMCA is an excellent example of a quality family gym. Besides a gym they have a pool, sports leagues, summer camps, child-care, and numerous other activities. They also provide financial assistance if needed to make sure everyone can afford to join.

If you do not have a local "Y" in your area look for a gym with similar characteristics. Most gyms will let you try them out a few times before making the decision join. Make sure you ask to see a list of their programs and classes. A good family gym should offer much more than a room full of exercise equipment!

The key to getting fit and staying fit is consistency. Get out and get moving as a family for an agreed upon amount of time every day, preferably at the same time. Keep your family's fitness routine simple during the work week, and save the more exciting physical endeavors for the weekends. Besides the obvious physical benefits you will grow closer as a family as well.

Chapter 9

The Usual Suspects

"In general my children refuse to eat anything
that hasn't danced on television."

-Erma Bombeck

Much of the blame for the unfit state of our
young people is put on the television and video
games. The TV and games themselves are not the
problem, rather it is the excessive amount of time
spent in front of them that is the problem. It is
important for children to learn the concept of

moderation. Too much of anything, good or bad, is usually not healthy.

If you vilify the things your children enjoy like television and video games you will probably put them on the defensive and at odds with the changes you are trying to implement. Instead set limits and purpose to have activities planned to take the place of the time they usually spend doing more sedentary activities. Most children sit in front of the TV out of habit or because they think they have nothing else to do...even if they have a million toys in their room.

In the early stages of weaning your children off of their electronics you will definitely meet with some resistance. You must come up with a workable plan and stick with it. The American Academy for Pediatrics recommends no more than 1-2 hours of TV per day, so this is a good guideline to go by.

There are a few ways to manage the TV. Some families give their children a daily time limit and let them choose what to watch and when to watch it. A modified version of this is to have a 'no television before an agreed upon time' policy. Another option is to choose a show or movie to watch together as a family in the evenings.

If your children are used to the television always being on then make sure to provide a lot of alternate activities like puzzles, coloring books, blocks, Legos, games, books, magazines and toys in your family room as well. This will encourage your child to do something else while they are watching TV and keep them from viewing the family room as the TV room.

Turn the TV off while you eat meals and snacks. Eating while watching the television often causes children to eat more at mealtime, as they are not paying attention to their food intake.

Snacking in front of the television has the same effect. Children who are used to eating snacks in front of the TV will often eat out of habit rather than hunger when watching television.

Experts highly recommended that you remove TV's from your children's rooms or at least make it off limits at bed time. An extensive study on sleep done by the Departments of Pediatrics and Child Family Psychology found that a child's daytime and nighttime viewing habits contributed to the greatest number of sleep disturbances.

Television in the bedroom was the greatest predictors of sleep problems. The more television a child viewed in a day the greater their difficulty falling and remaining asleep. In addition children who fall asleep watching TV often are stimulated to stay awake much longer than they would in a quiet room, therefore loosing valuable sleep.

(Ownes & Maxim Rolanda, 1999). Lack of sleep, in turn, has a negative effect on their health and nutrition.

CHAPTER 10

Ready...Set...

"It is impossible to win the race unless you venture to run, impossible to win the victory unless you dare to battle."

Richard M. Devos

There are several things to keep in mind before you take the family outside and try to get everyone to run for ten miles. If anyone in your family has any health problems or is significantly over weight please talk to your family doctor before beginning any exercise program. It would not be a bad idea to have sports physicals done on everybody before beginning any new exercise routine, even if your family is already in relatively good shape. Talk to your doctor about any concerns you have at this time as well.

Once your doctor has given your family the all clear you can get started. The first step is to buy the proper equipment you will need for the fitness activities your family has decided to pursue. You must have the proper shoes and safety equipment before you begin. You do not have to go out and purchase a hundred dollar pair of sneakers, but you does need to make sure everyone has shoes that they are comfortable in and that provide the proper amount of support. Good shoes will make exercise more comfortable and prevent long-term injuries down the road.

Make sure everyone has the proper safety equipment as well. Check your local laws to make sure you are aware of the local requirements for bikes and anything else you will be using. Personal reflective gear is important if you will be out walking, running, or biking later in the evening or early in the morning.

Proper hydration starts way before exercising. The amount of water the body needs depends on the temperature, intensity of the exercise, and individual weight. It is recommended that everyone consistently drink several glasses of water a day, and in addition always have water available while exercising. It is helpful if everyone has their own water bottle since they are more likely to drink more if it is convenient. Make sure to schedule frequent water breaks when exercising to insure your children are drinking an appropriate amount of water.

Although water hydrates quicker, sports drinks are acceptable to drink during exercise as well. They provide calories for an energy boost and help to keep electrolytes in balance. Since they taste good, children will usually drink more than if given plain water which is important since children are more susceptible to dehydration than adults. They have a lower sweat rate as well as less tolerance for extreme temperatures. (Healthy Living Staff, 2009)

Thirst is a sign of dehydration, so teach your children not to wait until their body cues them to drink. Watch for any signs of dehydration as you exercise. Signs of dehydration are:

- Increased heart rate
- Increased respiration
- Decreased sweating
- Decreased urination
- Sleepiness or tiredness
- Increased body temperature
- Extreme fatigue
- Muscle weakness or cramps
- Headaches, dizziness, or lightheadedness
- Nausea
- Tingling of the limbs

CAUTION: If dehydration is not caught in time it can quickly escalate. If your child displays any of the following symptoms they need immediate help. Please call an ambulance right away. Symptoms of severe dehydration include:

- Muscle spasms
- Vomiting
- Racing pulse
- Shriveled skin
- Dim vision
- Painful urination
- Confusion
- Difficulty breathing
- Seizures
- Chest and Abdominal pain
- Unconsciousness

Safety Note: Although rare, there is a danger in drinking too much water as well. Hyponatremia is caused by water intoxication and can be deadly. It is usually caused by drinking an extremely large amount of water in a short period of time. It is important to space your water intake throughout the day.

Before doing any physical activity make sure your family warms-up and stretches thoroughly. It is recommended that you spend at least 5-7 minutes stretching before to get your body ready to exercise. You want to stretch just until you can feel it and then hold the stretch between 20 and 30 seconds for the maximum benefit. Each stretch should be done in sets of three. It might be helpful to purchase a video that demonstrates proper stretching techniques until your family is comfortable doing them on their own.

It is important to insure your family takes the time to cool down after they are finished exercising as well. Have your family walk around slowly and stretch to help get their heart rate and blood pressure back to normal.

Chapter 11

...and GO!

"Motivation is what gets you started,

Habit is what keeps you going."

-Jim Rohn

There are four main types of exercise:
strength and resistance training, flexibility
exercise, endurance exercise, and balance and
coordination. Your best bet is to do a mixture of
the four. Your family should start and end each
exercise session with 5-10 minutes of flexibility i.e.
stretching exercises and then do some balance
and coordination work as a warm up. Then do

either resistance or endurance training for the rest of your time. It is good to alternate days, resistance one day and endurance the next, to provide your muscles time to rest and build up.

How competitive you make things depends greatly on your family dynamics. Fun competition might motivate some families, while it might spoil things for others. If that is the case teach your children how to compete against themselves and make a point to celebrate each other's victories.

You do not need to purchase exercise equipment unless you choose to do so. If you decide to purchase weights or machines check your local want ads before buying anything new. There is always a long list of gently and barely used exercise equipment for sale for a fraction of the price.

You may also consider buying a few fun DVD's if your family will be working out in the home or for snowy and rainy days. Pilates, Yoga, and Tai Chi, are all fun alternatives to the traditional workout and very effective. Yoga and Tai Chi are also excellent for stress relief.

While pricey, The Nintendo Wii offers a great workout program called *Wii Fit* that is fun for the whole family and tracks everyone's progress. It even allows you to set personal goals. The only drawback is only one person at a time can do it. The positive is that the rest of the family can have fun and encourage each other while awaiting their turn.

Strength and Resistance Exercises

Strength and resistance exercises focus on building muscle and improving bone strength by the use of resistance. (Martin) (This is not the same as body building or weight lifting.) This is great if anyone in your family suffers from muscle pain in a specific area like their back. By strengthening muscles most pain is alleviated. Strength and resistance training will also help your family prevent injuries. By strengthening the muscle groups they are less likely to be injured while working out or playing. Experts recommend strength and resistance training be done 3X a week for 20 minutes.

All your family needs to do resistance training is their own bodies. Exercise machines and free weights can also be used. If your family has decided to join a gym then they will train you on how to properly use these and set up an exercise program. If you are working out at home then it is best to build up your strength using your own body first to help prevent injuries. Exercises like pushups and crunches are examples of resistance training. Pilates is offered at most gyms and is a very effective form of resistance training.

Flexibility exercises

Flexibility exercises will improve the range of motion of your joints and muscles and increase blood flow. Stretching helps reduce your risk of injury when doing more strenuous exercise. Flexibility exercises should be done for at least 10 minutes a day and always before and after any physical activity. You will want teach your children to hold each stretch between 15-30 seconds taking care not to bounce which can cause injury. Exercises like stretching and Yoga are all great ways to improve flexibility. Most gyms offer Yoga classes. There are many kids Yoga tapes that are a lot of fun and a great workout for adults as well.

Endurance Exercises

Endurance or stamina exercises increase cardiovascular health and strength. The key to endurance exercises is sustained activity. Any activity that gets your heart rate up and your body moving will do. This form of exercise is the best for weight loss and for your heart. This is also the most fun form of exercise!

Depending on how fit your family currently is you can start with walking for a set amount of time daily until you build everyone's endurance up a little bit! To make walking more fun for your children make up scavenger hunt lists of things for them to try to spy on the walks. This will keep them busy and keep complaining to a minimum. Be creative and silly with the lists! Have small prizes for the daily winner. Your children might enjoy making lists as well once they have the hang of it.

Your family can take up traditional cardio exercises like biking, swimming, running, or aerobics. On the weekends you can also try some different activities like hockey, kayaking, mountain biking, or hiking. The goal is for children to associate exercise with fun, so pick things they will enjoy. If your children are older consider joining a club or team as a family that fits your interests. For example, a bicycle team or a hiking club.

For indoor workouts treadmills and elliptical trainers are great, but are not something the whole family can do together. Consider having everyone sign up for a daily time on these if you do get one.

Balance and Coordination Exercises

Balance and coordination exercises do just what they say for your body. They help you gain balance and coordination. Good coordination consists of balance, rhythm, spatial orientation, and the ability to quickly react to auditory and visual stimulus. (Grasso, 2010) Children often work on these as part of other sports or activities, but they can be worked on directly as well.

One of the best ways to work on balance and coordination as a family is to set up weekly obstacle courses in the back yard. Buy 10 small plastic signs, like a yard sale sign or for rent sign and number them 1-10. Write a different activity on the back of each with a dry erase marker. These signs wipe off easily so they can be reused again and again. For example: Jump rope 20 times, climb up slide, go across monkey bars with your eyes closed, do 10 crunches, slide down slip and slide 2 times etc. Then set the signs up in order around the yard. You can time each family member as they complete the obstacle course and record their times. Let your children design obstacle courses as well once they understand how to do it.

Organized sports or dance classes are great if your child is interested in them and your family has the time to make the commitment. There are competitive and non-competitive leagues depending on the personality of your child.

Make sure to respect what your child is, or is not, interested in and let their interests, not yours, drive their choices. For some children organized sports are fun and they love the sense of purpose and camaraderie. For other children organized sports are terrifying or overwhelming and they feel awkward. Some children prefer individual sports like Tae-Kwon Do or golf. Let your child's personality be your guide on this one.

If you have a fenced backyard stock it full of outdoor activities to encourage your children to get outside and move. You can set up a trampoline, volleyball or badminton net, horseshoe court, bocce ball court, croquet set, basketball hoop, etc. If you have younger children provide jump ropes and hula hoops as well. When weather permits, go outside as a family every night after dinner and play for awhile! Buy a cheap trophy and let the day's winner keep it in their room for the night to make things more fun.

The above information is just a guide to help you make some choices about how to incorporate fitness into your family's life. It is not so much important what you do, but rather that you get out and do something together as a family every day.

Chapter 12

Your Child's Body

"Beauty is the light in the heart."

-Kahil Gibran

With your family's new focus on fitness and nutrition it is important that your children understand your goal is that they feel good and that their bodies are healthy. Help them to think of their body as a machine that needs exercise and good food to run efficiently.

Tell your children they are perfectly and wonderfully made, so they do not feel like they need to be a certain size or shape to be healthy or attractive. Make sure to reiterate this often and be careful not to make any negative comments about their bodies, even if you are just joking or teasing.

It is difficult to teach them to love their bodies just as they are when every commercial and magazine out there tells them different. Did you know the majority fashion models are thinner than 98% of American Women? (NEDA, 2010) Try to avoid keeping magazines lying around or watching shows that glorify unrealistic body types. When the issue does arise, talk with your kids about it and how what they see and hear makes them feel. Explain that they cannot let their body image be controlled by outside sources or they will never be satisfied.

Even good things can be overdone. Watch your child for any signs of compulsion or an unnatural focus on their body, their weight, or exercising. If you notice anything that concerns you take action immediately. Of the 8 million people with eating disorders Ninety-five percent are between the ages of 11 and 25. Even though girls are more likely to have an eating disorder they affect boys as well. Eating disorders are serious and can quickly become deadly. Do not try to handle it alone, but seek professional help.

Chapter 13

Special Considerations

A human being is a single being.

Unique and unrepeatable.

-Eileen Caddy

While this book was meant as a general overview of fitness and nutrition for all families, every family reading this is unique. If you have a child with health problems or special needs do not let it scare you away from exercise, rather let it inspire you to find alternate ways to get fit as a whole family. Talk with your doctor about the best way to involve everyone.

Design activities that meet the medical needs of the whole family as much as possible. If you or one of your children has to do daily physical or occupational therapy exercises then get everyone involved. The whole family can do the exercises with them before going on with the other planned fitness activities.

If there are some activities one of your children cannot participate in or that and cannot be modified to fit their needs find another way to involve them. Let them set up the game, be the referee , blow the whistle, put them in charge of the stop watch, keeping score, keeping statistics on family members or anything else they will enjoy doing.

If you have a child with very limited movement or a chronic illness that makes exercise impossible, ask them to be the family sports photographer or reporter. Have them journal, take pictures or video tape the day's fitness activities.

Teach them how to put everything on the computer and edit to create a weekly family fitness highlight video or slide show set to the music of their choice. Remember this is a family endeavor so insist that everyone be involved to the best of their ability and be supportive of one another.

Final Note

The journey towards a fitter and healthier family is not an easy one. When there are setbacks, accept them as such and start again. When there are tears, meet them with acceptance and encouragement.

If your family stays consistent you will see such a difference in everyone's health, energy level, and self confidence this time next year. I assure you it will be well worth the effort.

It is our hope that the activities in this book bring you closer together as a family as you laugh, sweat, and cook healthy meals together! Above all....have fun!

Recipes

Quick and Tasty Breakfasts

Breakfast is truly the most important meal of the day, so don't let your children skip it. Breakfast can be tricky since mornings are often so rushed. For extra early mornings you can make muffins the night before! Just warm them up and add fruit or a yogurt the next morning. You can also keep pancake and waffle batter mixed and in the fridge so all you have to do is pour and cook. The following ideas take less than 5 minutes to make, and are delicious as well as healthy.

Whole Wheat Instant Waffles: smother in fruit and drizzle with honey or spread with Nutella

Breakfast Burrito Wraps: scramble eggs and add chopped ham or reduced fat crumbled bacon, cilantro, and a pinch of shredded cheese. Add salsa and wrap up in a whole wheat tortilla.

Parfait: Layer all natural vanilla yogurt with granola and fresh fruit.

Cottage cheese: Add sliced peaches and wholegrain toast.

Cereal: There is nothing wrong with cereal for breakfast as long it is of the healthy variety!

English Muffins: Whole Wheat English Muffins with peanut butter or one of the alternatives and some all fruit spread will give your child a great boost of energy!

The following recipes are quick and easy as well. Make the muffins and the pancake batter the night before to save valuable time in the morning.

Apple Oatmeal:

- 1 cup water
- 1/4 cup apple juice or applesauce
- 1 apple, cored and chopped
- 2/3 cup rolled oats
- 1 teaspoon ground cinnamon
- 1 cup milk

Directions

1. Combine the water, apple juice, and apples in a saucepan. Bring to a boil over high heat, and stir in the rolled oats and cinnamon. Return to a boil, then reduce heat to low, and simmer until thick, about 3 minutes. Spoon into serving bowls, and pour milk over the servings.

Eggs in a Basket

- whole wheat bread
- 1 Tbsp. butter
- large eggs
- kosher salt and pepper to taste

Directions:

1. Heat an electric griddle to 350 degrees or heat a large frying pan over medium-high heat.
2. Place 1 teaspoon of butter on the griddle.
3. Use a cookie cutter to cut out your favorite shape in the center of each piece of bread.
4. Butter one side of each piece of bread, including the cutout pieces, with the remaining butter.
5. Place the bread, butter side down on the griddle.
6. Break one egg into a small dish. Gently slide it into the hole of one of the bread slices.
7. Repeat with the remaining eggs and bread slices.
8. Cook until the egg is golden on the bottom, a minute or two. Gently flip to cook on the other side, about 1 minute.
9. Flip the cutout pieces of toast to cook on the other side until toasted, another minute or so.

Morning Glory Muffins

- 2 cups all-purpose flour
- 1 1/4 cups white sugar
- 2 teaspoons baking soda
- 2 teaspoons ground cinnamon
- 1/4 teaspoon salt
- 2 cups shredded carrots
- 1/2 cup raisins
- 1/2 cup chopped walnuts
- 1/2 cup unsweetened flaked coconut
- 1 apple - peeled, cored and shredded
- 3 eggs
- 1 cup vegetable oil
- 2 teaspoons vanilla extract

Directions

1. Preheat oven to 350 degrees F (175 degrees C). Grease 12 muffin cups, or line with paper muffin liners.
2. In a large bowl, mix together flour, sugar, baking soda, cinnamon, and salt. Stir in the carrot, raisins, nuts, coconut, and apple.
3. In a separate bowl, beat together eggs, oil, and vanilla. Stir egg mixture into the carrot/flour mixture, just until moistened. Scoop batter into prepared muffin cups.
4. Bake in preheated oven for 20 minutes, until a toothpick inserted into center of a muffin comes out clean.

Pumpkin Pancakes

- 2 cups all-purpose flour
- 3 tablespoons brown sugar
- 2 teaspoons baking powder
- 1 teaspoon baking soda
- 1 teaspoon ground allspice
- 1 teaspoon ground cinnamon
- 1/2 teaspoon ground ginger
- 1/2 teaspoon salt
- 1 1/2 cups milk
- 1 cup pumpkin puree
- 1 egg
- 2 tablespoons vegetable oil
- 2 tablespoons vinegar

Directions

1. In a separate bowl, mix together the milk, pumpkin, egg, oil and vinegar. Combine the flour, brown sugar, baking powder, baking soda, allspice, cinnamon, ginger and salt, stir into the pumpkin mixture just enough to combine.
2. Heat a lightly oiled griddle or frying pan over medium high heat. Pour or scoop the batter onto the griddle, using approximately 1/4 cup for each pancake. Brown on both sides and serve hot.

Applesauce Pancakes

- 2 cups dry pancake mix (not a "just add water" mix)
- 1 teaspoon ground cinnamon
- 2 eggs
- 1 cup applesauce
- 1 teaspoon lemon juice
- 1/2 cup milk

Directions

1. In a large bowl, stir together pancake mix and cinnamon. Make a well in the center of the pancake mix. Add the eggs, applesauce, lemon juice and milk; stir until smooth.
2. Heat a lightly oiled griddle or frying pan over medium high heat. Pour or scoop the batter onto the griddle, using approximately 1/4 cup for each pancake. Brown on both sides and serve hot.

Smoothies

Smoothies are quick, delicious, and nutritious way to start the day or hold your child over until their next meal. They are rich in calcium rich and a fun way to get them to eat fruit. All you need to keep on hand is vanilla yogurt, ice, juice, and a few bags of various frozen fruits. You can also add some honey for extra sweetness if you need too. There are a million different smoothie recipes out there and I am sure you and your family will enjoy creating your own as well. Here are a few to get you started.

Lemon Blueberry Smoothie

- 1 cup frozen blueberries
- 1/2 cup frozen pineapple chunks
- 1 cup low-fat milk
- 1 Tbsp. frozen lemonade concentrate
- 1/2 cup vanilla yogurt
- 1 Tbsp. honey (optional)

Directions:

1. Place the blueberries and pineapple chunks in a blender or food processor.
2. Pour milk in next. Add remaining ingredients.
3. Puree until smooth, stopping to press fruit into the blades of the blender, if necessary.

Strawberry Banana Smoothies

- 1-1/2 cups frozen sliced strawberries (or fresh strawberries)
- 1 banana
- 1 Tbsp. orange juice concentrate
- 1 cup milk
- 1/2 cup ice, if using fresh strawberries instead of frozen
- ½ cup vanilla yogurt

Directions:

1. Place strawberries and banana in a blender. If using fresh strawberries in place of frozen, add ice at this point.
2. Top with orange juice concentrate and milk.
3. Puree until smooth.

Orange Smoothies

- 1 11 oz. can mandarin oranges in juice
- 1/2 cup frozen pineapple chunks
- 1/2 cup vanilla yogurt
- 1 Tbsp. honey
- 1 cup milk
- 1/2 cup ice

Directions:

1. Open can of oranges and drain. Place in a zip-top plastic bag and freeze several hours.
2. Place the frozen oranges and pineapple chunks in the bottom of a blender.
3. Puree until the mixture reaches the texture of a milkshake. Add more ice, if desired, until an icy consistency is achieved.

Power Packed Lunches

For lunch you want to stick with a pretty standard formula. Your child's can greatly impact the rest of their school day. The following spread will help them stay alert in class and keep them from feeling sluggish: a healthy drink, a balanced anchor, a fruit, a vegetable, and a healthy snack. Make sure to stay away from anything high in sugar, refined carbohydrates, excess sodium or trans fats.

Healthy Drinks

The following drinks are nutritious and satisfying to young taste buds: White milk, lightly sweetened iced tea, 100 percent fruit and/or vegetable drinks. While it is difficult to get most children to drink a straight vegetable drink there are several drinks that offer a full serving of fruits and vegetables that taste just like a fruit drink. Tea is packed with antioxidants. Experiment with all different kinds and flavor with a small amount of sugar, honey, or agave nectar.

A Balanced Anchor

Sandwiches do not have to be traditional! Instead of white bread choose one of the following whole wheat alternatives: rounds, English muffins, pita bread, wraps, tortillas, bagels and crackers. Provide a lean meat like turkey or ham and fresh cheese. The traditional cheeses like cheddar and Colby are fine, but don't be afraid to experiment...asiago, baby swiss, havarti, etc. Your child may find a new favorite! If they will eat it add veggies to their sandwiches as well. Flavored cream cheese is a yummy alternative to mayonnaise.

Peanut butter and Jelly are always a favorite. Your child may also like almond butter, cashew butter, hazelnut butter, soy butter, or sunflower butter. Most Jelly is high in sugar and high fructose corn syrup, so opt for all fruit spreads with no added sugar or apple butter instead.

CAUTION: If your child is allergic to peanut butter they may very well be allergic to other nuts as well. Please talk to your child's allergist before trying any of the alternatives.

Soup, pasta and sauce or flavored Asian noodles are also good, especially on cold days. Look at the labels closely and find one with the best ingredients and least sodium. Sodium content is often through the roof on instant foods like these.

Fruits & Vegetables

Vegetables

Slice up raw vegetables like peppers, cucumber, carrots, squash, and zucchini for easy eating. Raw green beans, banana peppers, and snap peas are delicious too, and can be eaten as is. If your child will only eat their veggies with ranch dressing, look for one that is low in fat.

Fruit

Any fruit is fine for lunch. You may also want to put a fruit salad in their lunch with an array of different colored fruit. Try any mix of the following kiwi, cantaloupe, banana, apples, blueberries, oranges, nectarines, peaches, blackberries, raspberries, strawberries, grapes, mango, papaya, pineapple, star fruit, and watermelon.

Snacks

It is always nice to end a meal with something sweet. Homemade trail mix with dark chocolate, granola bars, yogurt or yogurt drink, graham crackers with Nutella spread, rice crispy treats, pudding, teddy grahams, and Jell-O are all fairly healthy choices for snacks.

Super Snacks

Snacks can be healthy and fun! Here are some quick ideas that don't require any cooking to keep your children going between meals.

Healthy Substitutions

Chips: crackers, tortilla chips, mini-rice cakes, carrots, and celery.

Healthy Dips: humus, bean dip, salsa, yogurt, Nutella, peanut butter, and guacamole.

Silly Faces: Give your child a rice cake with peanut butter or cream cheese spread on top of it. Let them make a face with chopped up fruit and vegetables. Sprouts make great hair!

Snack Kabobs: Give each child a skewer (for younger children use coffee stirrers) Let them put bite sized pieces of fruit and cheese on it and make their own snack kabobs.

Sandwich on a Stick: Give each child a skewer (for younger children use coffee stirrers)   Provide your child with a plate of cubed bread, cheese, chicken breast or ham, cucumber and cherry tomatoes. Let your children put together their "sandwiches."

Fruit Burritos: Spread peanut butter on a flour tortilla. Add bananas, strawberries, peaches, and blueberries or any fruit of your liking. Drizzle with vanilla yogurt. Roll and eat!

Fish Pond: Put a small amount of blue dye in cream cheese. Mix and spread it onto a plate. Sprinkle whole wheat gold fish into the "pond". Let your children use pretzel fishing poles to catch their fish. They can use the cream cheese to make the fish stick to their poles.

Ant Farm: Spread a plate with peanut butter. Erect a tunnel using graham crackers. Place the raisins on the peanut butter to look like ants. Let your children use the graham crackers to scoop up the 'ants' and peanut butter!

Frozen Banana Pops

Cut a banana in half an insert a popsicle stick. Place them in the freezer on wax paper for about 10 minutes. Crush granola, cereal, or graham crackers. Remove the banana from the freezer, coat with peanut butter, and let the children dip it in the mixture.

Cut a banana in half an insert a popsicle stick. Dip the bananas in yogurt and roll in chopped nuts, coconut shavings and crushed cereal. Place them in the freezer on wax paper for about 1 hour. Remove the banana from the freezer and eat.

Mini-Pizzas: Split a whole wheat English muffin in half. Spread with tomato sauce and shredded part-skim mozzarella cheese. Bake in the oven for about 10 minutes at 350 degrees.

Fruit Salad Cones: Mix a cup of yogurt with a sliced banana, a can of drained mandarin oranges, drained pineapple chunks and just a few mini-marshmallows. Spoon into ice cream cones.

Healthy Snack Mixes

Energy bars and trail mixes are great to make in large batches to snack on throughout the week.

Energy Bars

Awesome Energy Bars

1/2 cup peanut butter

1/4 cup margarine

1 bag miniature marshmallows

2 1/2 cups Cheerios

1 1/2 cups Rice Krispies

1/2 cup raisins

1/2 cup peanuts

1/2 cup chocolate chips

Melt peanut butter, margarine and marshmallows in microwave.

Place cereals, raisins, peanuts in large bowl. Stir in peanut butter mixture and mix all together. Press into a lightly buttered 13 x 9-inch pan. Let cool and then cut into bars.

Trekking Energy Bars

- 2 cups whole wheat flour
- 1 cup unsweetened flaked coconut
- 1/2 cup sesame seed
- 1/2 cup pumpkin seeds
- 1/2 cup sunflower seed
- 1/2 cup flax seed
- 3/4 cup raisins
- 1/2 cup dark chocolate chips
- 1 1/2 cups natural-style peanut butter
- 1 cup applesauce
- ½ cup of honey
- 1 teaspoon vanilla extract

Directions

1. Preheat oven to 350.

2. Mix all dry ingredients together.

3. Add peanut butter, honey, and vanilla - mix well. (I used my mixer - it's pretty dense).

4. Grease a 13x9 baking pan - spread mixture into pan (should be about an inch thick).

5. Bake for 15-20 minutes.

6. Cool and cut into squares.

Simple & Delicious Energy Bars

- 1 cup natural-style peanut butter
- 1 cup honey
- 3 cups dry uncooked old-fashioned oatmeal

Directions

1. Combine peanut butter and honey in a large nonstick pot and warm up over a low heat until runny and mixed.
2. Mix in the oatmeal.
3. You don't want to cook it, just heat it up enough to stir everything together nicely.
4. Press into a 9x9-inch pan.
5. Let cool, then cut into 16 equal bars.
6. Wrap each bar in foil and store in plastic bags. - No need to refrigerate as the ingredients are natural.

Monkey Chow Bar

- 1 cup peanut butter
- 1/2 cup honey
- 1/4 teaspoon vanilla extract
- 1/3 cup sunflower seed
- 2/3 cup dried cherries or dried cranberries or raisins (or a combination)
- 3 tablespoons sesame seeds

- 1/3 cup shredded coconut
- 3 cups puffed brown rice cereal
- butter, to grease pan
- Dark chocolate or carob chips
- Sliced almonds

Directions

1. Grease an 8x8 pan with a little butter.
2. In a large bowl, mix together the peanut butter, honey and vanilla extract until well-combined.
3. Add the sunflower seeds, dried fruit, sesame seeds and coconut and combine thoroughly with the peanut butter mixture.
4. Gradually add the puffed brown rice cereal to this.
5. Mix everything together.
6. Firmly press the mixture into the prepared 8x8 pan; you'll need to wet your hands

slightly, otherwise the mixture just sticks to them.

7. Cover and refrigerate for a couple of hours, then cut and serve.

Trail Mixes

It is easy to make trail mixes with whatever you have in the pantry. Most will keep well in an airtight container. Any mix of the following will work well:

> Cereal, granola, popcorn
>
> Nuts of all kinds
>
> Any variety or a mixture of dried fruits
>
> Sunflower seeds or pumpkin seeds
>
> Animal crackers, teddy grahams, goldfish
>
> Dark chocolate pieces

Cranberry Raisin Trail Mix

- 1/2 cup butter or margarine

- 1/3 cup honey
- 1/4 cup packed brown sugar
- 1 teaspoon ground cinnamon
- 1/2 teaspoon salt
- 3 cups square oat cereal
- 1 1/2 cups old-fashioned oats
- 1 cup chopped walnuts
- 1/2 cup dried cranberries
- 1/2 cup chocolate-covered raisins

Directions

1. In a saucepan or microwave-safe bowl, combine the first five ingredients; heat until the butter is melted. Stir until the sugar is dissolved.
2. In a large bowl, combine cereal, oats and nuts. Drizzle with butter mixture and mix well. Place in a greased 15-in. x 10-in. x 1-in. baking pan. Bake, uncovered, at 275 degrees F for 45 minutes, stirring every 15

minutes. Cool for 15 minutes, stirring occasionally. Stir in cranberries and chocolate-covered raisins.

Nutty Trail Mix

- 3 cups oats (I use rolled oats)
- 1 1/2 cups wheat bran or oat bran
- 1 cup powdered milk
- 1 cup chopped pecans or walnuts
- 1/2 cup sesame seed
- 1/2 cup hulled sunflower seed
- 1/2 cup unsweetened flaked coconut
- 1/2 cup slivered almond
- 1 cup honey
- 1/4 cup vegetable oil
- 1/2 cup raisins
- 1/2 cup chopped dried apricot

Directions

1. Preheat oven to 300°F.

2. In a large mixing bowl, stir together oats, wheat bran, milk powder, pecans, sesame seeds, sunflower seeds, coconut and almonds.
3. In a 2-cup measure, stir together honey and oil until blended; pour over dry ingredients.
4. Using two spoons, toss and stir to combine well.
5. Turn onto lightly greased baking sheets; spreading evenly.
6. Bake 25 to 35 minutes or until golden brown, stirring every 10 minutes.
7. Immediately, turn into large bowl; stir in raisins and apricots.
8. Cool completely.
9. Store in an airtight container.

Granola Trail Mix

1 cup granola crunch cereal

1 cup yogurt raisins

1 cup craisens

1 cup peanuts

1 cup chocolate covered soy nuts

1/4 cup sunflower seeds (no shells)

1/4 mini marshmallows

Mix together in a big bowl and enjoy!

Kid Chow Trail Mix

3 c. Honey Nut Cheerios

3 c. Corn Chex

3 c. Rice Chex

2 c. pretzels, sm. size

2 c. raisins

1/2 c. coconut

Mix and toss all ingredients together.

Trail Mix with a Kick

1/2 c. butter

1 tbsp. Worcestershire sauce

1/2 tsp. seasoned salt

1 c. salted peanuts

2 c. pretzel sticks

2 c. mixed wheat, rice & corn cereal

2 c. popcorn

1 1/2 c. raisins

1 tsp. chili powder

Heat butter with Worcestershire sauce, chili powder, seasoned salt in large pan, stirring to combine. Add peanuts, pretzels and cereal squares. Mix gently. Spread on baking sheet and bake in 275 degree oven for 45 minutes. Stir after 15 minutes. After 30 minutes, add popcorn and raisins. Stir and bake 15 minutes longer.

Works Cited

Ansorage, R. (2010, February 23). *Excercise Found to Decrease Anxiety in Chronic Illness.* Retrieved April 29, 2010, from MentalHelp.net: http://www.mentalhelp.net/poc/view_doc.php?type=news&id=126141&cn=288

ASPE . (2002, June 20). *Physical Activity Fundamental To Preventing Disease*. Retrieved April 28, 2010, from ASPE.hhs.gov: http://aspe.hhs.gov/health/reports/physicalactivity /

Centers for Disease Control and Prevention. (2010, February 26). *Overweight and Obesity*. Retrieved April 27, 2010, from Centers for Disease Control and Prevention: http://www.cdc.gov/obesity/

David, S. (2000, March). *Diet and Behavior in Children*. Retrieved April 29, 2010, from Center for Science in the Public Interest: http://www.cspinet.org/nah/3_00/diet_behavior. html

Dean, J. (2010). *How Long to Form a Habit*. Retrieved May 1, 2010, from PSYBLOG: http://www.spring.org.uk/2009/09/how-long-to-form-a-habit.php

Division of Nutrition, Physical Activity, and Obesity. (2009, October 20). *Overweight and Obesity: Consequences*. Retrieved April 27, 2010, from Centers for Disease Control and Prevention:

http://www.cdc.gov/obesity/causes/economics.html

Food for the Brain Staff. (n.d.). *School Grades Success With Food For Thought.* Retrieved May 9, 2010, from Food For The Brain: http://www.foodforthebrain.org/content.asp?id_Content=1741

Fouad, T. M. (2004, April 5). *CDC: Obesity approaching tobacco as top preventable cause of death.* Retrieved April 27, 2010, from Doctor's Lounge: http://www.doctorslounge.com/primary/articles/obesity_death/

Grasso, B. Y. (2010). *Cordination & Movement Skill Development.* Retrieved May 11, 2010, from Perform Better: http://www.performbetter.com/catalog/matriarch/OnePiecePage.asp_Q_PageID_E_209_A_PageName_E_ArticleCoordMovement

Healthy Child Staff. (2010). *10 Reasons to Keep Kids Off Soda.* Retrieved May 8, 2010, from Healthy Child: http://www.healthychild.com/child-nutrition/10-reasons-to-keep-kids-off-soda/

Healthy Living Staff. (2009, May 04). *Sports Drinks VS. Water.* Retrieved May 5, 2010, from Healthy Living: http://www.healthy-living-best.com/healthy-eating/115-sports-drinks-vs-water

LiveScience Staff. (2009, November 4). *Unhealthy Food Ads Pervasive on Kids' Shows.* Retrieved April 27, 2009, from LiveScience: http://www.livescience.com/health/091104-kids-food-ads-tv.html

Martin, B. (n.d.). *Types of Excercise.* Retrieved May 11, 2010, from Improving Health and Energy: http://www.improving-health-and-energy.com/types-of-exercise.html

NEDA. (2010). *Statistics: Eating Disorders and their Precursors.* Retrieved May 9, 2010, from NationalEatingDisorders.org: http://www.nationaleatingdisorders.org/uploads/statistics_tmp.pdf

Nemours Foundation. (2010). *How TV Affects Your Child.* Retrieved April 28, 2010, from Kids Health : http://kidshealth.org/parent/positive/family/tv_affects_child.html

NSF Staff. (2009). *How Much Sleep Do We Really Need.* Retrieved April 29, 2010, from National Sleep Foundation: http://www.sleepfoundation.org/article/how-sleep-works/how-much-sleep-do-we-really-need

Ownes, J. M., & Maxim Rolanda, M. (1999, September 3). Television-viewing Habits and Sleep Disturbances in Children. *Pediatrics Vol. 104 No. 3* , p. e27.

Rabin, C. R. (2010, February 19). *Child Obestity Risks Death at Early Age, Study Finds.* Retrieved April 27, 2010, from The New York Times: http://www.nytimes.com/2010/02/11/health/11fat.html

Sloane, S. (2009, October 25). *Obesity: A Weighty Issue.* Retrieved April 27, 2010, from CBS News: http://www.cbsnews.com/stories/2009/10/25/sunday/main5419040.shtml

Wansink, B. P. (2008, March 7). *Stop when you're full? You must be French.* Retrieved May 8, 2010, from MSNBC: http://www.msnbc.msn.com/id/23449358/